Stay healthy with my vegetable diet

Your Body Will Thank You

Brittany Lazaro

Contents

Chapter One

INTRO

Like most People change plants, I was wondering if there is enough food. Also, I worry about finding an uninspired and restrictive vegetarian diet, I often find vegetarian food boring and mundane. Teaching him to cook healthy food on the floor isn't enough to teach him. I trained as a chef at Intuitive Vegetable Kitchen, where I learned to cook with the intuition of a chef. I wanted to make sure my body got everything it needed, so I went to school to learn about the nutrition I needed, focusing on a natural approach to a healthy lifestyle. I've never liked cooking and eating like this. I have never felt limited or closed. Instead, I'm obsessed with constantly adding new and interesting foods and dishes to my recipe list and exploring the endless possibilities with new flavors and flavor combinations. Since I switched to a plant-based lifestyle, I have more energy. I lost weight without trying. And I have no chronic gas or digestive problems. I had it until I recovered, I didn't realize how bad it was. This is how my plant-based journey evolved, but I know that every journey is different because our experiences with food are different. The way we eat is very individual. Food not only nourishes our bodies, it also has the power to make life happier. Food is closely linked to culture and social life and our taste buds assure us pleasure and satisfaction from eating. Leading a plant-based lifestyle is both difficult and easy for the entire community. Most people are afraid to give up food and learn to cook new and exotic dishes with people they don't know much about and sometimes can't even talk to. Eating plants isn't natural and it's hard to believe that plants are featured in countless vegan cookbooks and blogs. This is yet another book. The diet and recipes in this book are designed to teach you about the best plant food, so eating is encouragement. As for plants, add more vegetables to your diet, loss of loss, show this special ancient event, bring chronic changes in health, relief and symptoms of chronic or decreasing diseases, hiilijalanj v s he hnt s hnt s m s m s m s m s ll s' Yasa ; Indeed. I decided to practice cooking, but this dish was not far from success. Using the knowledge and techniques that have helped me and many of my clients, I have carefully crafted these recipes to quickly and easily discover a variety of foods. I am inspired by devices from all over the world, so I find a new food, a recipe or a favorite recipe and expand my vocabulary and my culinary experience. Plus, the three-week meal plan includes daily menus and grocery lists that show you exactly how to prepare these meals and help you stay on track. You will find clear guidance and a comprehensive approach plan for a complete vegan diet that is consistently dominated by tasty and healthy foods. You can also cook dishes that will delight meat lovers. After all, the best thing about enjoying herbs is that after three weeks you will start to see and feel their healing power. Your butt will look great, your digestion will improve, you'll have more energy, you'll think better, and you'll sleep better. If you follow this diet long enough, you should find that your immune sys-

tem is much stronger, your mood is more balanced, your life is lighter, and so is your mind.
calmer.   decisions.

Chapter Two

MY SECRETS

All Even if there are a lot of disagreements among nutritionists and physicians on what constitutes a WFPB diet, there is one thing they all agree on: a veggie or WFPB diet does more than simply help you lose weight. To begin with, it's a way of life for me.

A vegetarian diet may mean various things to different individuals. Some vegetarians eat dairy items like eggs and cheese, while others refuse to consume any animal products at all.

A SECRET TO LOSE WEIGHT WITHOUT CONSCIOUSNESS

Make Do with Bowls and Plates Most individuals tend to eat greater servings when they are served on a large dish or bowl because they want to fill the space. It's easier to control how much food you consume if your plates and bowls are the same size at each meal.

In order to keep things simple, stick to only two or three tastes. In order for us to feel satiated, we need to encounter a specific quantity of diverse flavors in our food. In order to ensure that everyone can enjoy the food, we need to limit the number of various dishes and tastes on the table at a given moment. A good example of this would be the T s s k s manual. The stuffing isn't even done when we cook a dinner made up of only two or three separate dishes.

Use a pair of chopsticks to eat. Because it slows us down and creates little bits, we are more likely to feel satisfied before we eat too much.

Between each mouthful, swallow. It's a lot more difficult than you may think! To see whether you're eating unconsciously, try paying attention to your jaw movements. In addition, it reduces the onset of fullness more slowly.

After each meal, brush your teeth. This is a terrific concept for oral hygiene and it also decreases the possibility of inadvertent eating between meals. Snacks that provide energy and nutrients are clearly beneficial, but it's preferable to avoid taking in more than is absolutely required.

Food Caloric Density Modification The caloric content of brown rice may be reduced by cooking it with an additional cup of water. There won't be any major difference. The morning is a good time to do this since it's simpler to mix and provides extra water to start the day.

Juice or soda may be diluted with water. Drinking more water instead of sugary drinks might help you shed a few pounds. When it comes to sugar, you may drink as much as 100 percent natural fruit juice and not realize how many calories you've consumed. Can't you just stop doing it? Drinks may be diluted with water or non-alcoholic beverages at the beginning of the process. Sugar consumption will be reduced if they are halved. Add a little amount of flavoring to sparkling water or gas and dilute it gradually.

Chapter Three

ADVICES

Plants, as well as other advantages

Many more health advantages may be gained by consuming a variety of plants. When moving to a herbal diet, these are some of the side effects that individuals have reported experiencing.

Swap out sugary and refined grains for more nutrient-dense vegetarian meals that give you energy. This will help keep your blood sugar levels under control.

It's important to keep your face clean since dairy products are a major cause of acne. Reducing your intake of refined sugars and switching to whole grain sweets will help clear your skin.

Enhanced Immune System Plants are great sources of the nutrients your immune system need. Focus on dark green, red, and orange fruits and vegetables, as well as zinc-rich seeds, such as pumpkin seeds.

Improved Absorption Many individuals report that their digestion improves when they eat a diet rich in fiber. I've had many customers tell me that since they had a smaller stomach, the trousers were better for them.

The s-section of the magical and the culprits s n s r s stykseen and ruoansulatush s iri ö in may be used to ease the stomach after eating too much meat, dairy, products, and fats.

Recovery time after workout is reduced. People that eat a portion of a plant-based diet that rapidly replenishes after exercising include athletes, runners, and bodybuilders.

Reduce the danger of catastrophic neurological illnesses, help the earth, and enjoy days sy lots of delicious and nutritious recipes if you can maintain a healthy lifestyle and eat a diet rich in herbs. Those who have a great sense of style: Who's still keeping you from changing?

It's not clear whether the food will be any better than it used to be.

Be assured, a vegetarian diet is not the only option available when it comes to eating veggies (although leafy vegetables are quite important). There are occasions when the same veggies are not able to supply enough smokers to boost performance.

It's a mix of things.

Bananas and a wide variety of other fruits and vegetables. As it turns out, this is also one of your favorite fruits.

• Vegetables such as carrots, lettuce, cabbage, broccoli, and cabbage may also be included to this list.

• Whole grains including barley, millet, oats, wheat, and quinoa.

This includes legumes like lentils, chick peas and black beans.

It is possible to transform tubers like potatoes and maize, as well as peas and other vegetables, into delectable dishes.

When it comes to food, you'll be amazed at the diversity of cuisines, desserts, and even healthful foods like fire. Even if you had to give up certain suosikkiruoista and snacks, I can say that s meals EIV s t would be boring HCl or uninteresting HCl.

More often than not, the amylaceouos concentrates on foods that have relied on it for centuries and are still reliant on it now.

You may create goods such as black beans and maize as well as peas and potatoes in addition to brown rice and quinoa. Most of these items are familiar to you, but they may be cooked differently than you are used to, so feel free to include them in your meals. You may have as much of the sweet potato lasagna, mashed potatoes, and salsa as you want, as well as the black beans and rice burrito.

You don't have to worry about calorie tracking or dosage management when you consume vegetarian meals since you can freely express your preferences. With more fiber and water, the volume in vegetarian diets takes up more space in the stomach than in a traditional burger, which consequently fills the stomach and eliminates hunger, even if you've eaten less food.

Some individuals who follow this diet worry about consuming some form of green vegetables, calcium, beans for protein, or nuts for fat; you have to give up that thinking, since the key to this lifestyle is the choice of food for the full plant you want to consume.

Many everyday items, such as burgers, potatoes, and fast food, will be invented within a short period of time.

Can you continue to live this way?

There is no doubt in my mind that you are correct. My response to the question has always been and will remain the same.

The body benefits from minimizing refined and processed meals, such as ordering your favorite items and substituting herbs, according to experts.

To begin a herbal diet, you will experience immediate effects like lower blood pressure, lower cholesterol, less medication use, improved sleep at night, and even the capacity to wear old clothing. Become!

However, you're unsure of how to keep yourself inspired to keep going. If you're not satisfied with the results you're getting and you're beginning to overcome roadblocks, you should know that there are various paths you may take to achieve a healthy lifestyle.

There are a variety of methods to live this lifestyle, including the following:

First and foremost, be your own best source of inspiration.

It is possible to live this lifestyle as an assistant and to motivate yourself to reach your objectives. Set up the records and begin the decryption process on your own. Consider, for example, the scenario where you wish to run a whole marathon without running out of breath while dressed in old clothes or a certain size. This award-winning magazine and movie may be saved. Notes written by me may also be read at a later time to encourage him or to provide updates on his progress.

2. Allow people to serve as sources of inspiration for you.

If achievement isn't enough to motivate you, look for someone who can. To keep you motivated, you may watch videos of individuals who have successfully lost weight and share their stories.

Learn from others' experiences. It's a great way to keep on track and inspired.

Three. Never stop learning

Consult books on healthy diet, natural cooking, professional advice, or nutritionists' recommen-dations, such as this one. You may take a step forward in the correct way by learning something new about this lifestyle and getting advise on what you're doing well and wrong and how to do it better. Reading helps you stay on top of your workload since it offers you a sense of empower-ment.

The fourth step is to be inventive.

There are moments when eating is the only thing keeping you going. Use a shopping list or chilled content to construct what you want. You won't have a hard time following a vegetable-based diet. What do you think? This is the way to achieve success, pleasure, and self-worth (I have a recipe department in this book, so keep reading).

5. Join an online support group.

Keep in mind that you are not the only one in this situation; someone else has discovered what you have and managed to live. In spite of the fact that your loved ones don't believe in your decision, there are a plethora of online lifestyle groups where members share their tales, fights with food, recipes, and more.

Drop the vehicle off, but don't leave it there; do it and then come back.

Is Eating a Plant-Based Diet Expensive?

In fact, a high-vegetable and all-products diet might cost you as little as $ 3 a day! To be clear, you read it right. I'm not referring to all of the meals of the day; rather, I'm referring to DAY food, which is on par with other meals in terms of nutritional value. It's a lot cheaper than eating out or buying food, even if you prepare it yourself.

Furthermore, it enjoys better and more nutritious meals, and it spends less than a third of what it would have originally spent on food.

Some individuals mistakenly believe that a plant-based diet consists only of salads, rather than the whole spectrum of foods available to an-imals. It's tough to stick to a diet for an extended period of time if you're terrified of it or feel bad about it being focused exclusively on your own personal health. Many of my customers come to me because they've tried using plants but have become so sick of them that they need assistance keeping things in check.

Even though I don't believe oils and sweets to be particularly healthy, they may serve a purpose if they're utilized in moderation to improve flavor and encourage long-term healthy eating. To generate money, the bank would want to see customers eat more pumpkins than carrots. The lack of health and taste in bed go hand in hand, and that's why I'd want a lot of attention after that. Improved global health and less animal suffering may go hand in hand with the desire to better one's own well-being. Trifecta, it turns out, might help you stay motivated, making it a lifestyle rather than a diet.

As a first impression, many individuals believe that herbal diets are very rigid and excessive. Is it possible to have a bed with a greater range of goods on the bed that yel these colors? Is it possible to have a bed with a greater variety of products on the bed that yel these colors? agricultural kt yellow Coles More pleasant this time, the mind hears the voices of its chefs. Since the beginning, I've been immersed in an intriguing and flavorful new universe, free of boundaries or restrictions. I'd want to expose you to the fascinating world of plants you've discovered.

When it comes to a healthy diet, there is no better place to start than with vegetables. Included here are all of the plant parts indicated above, including leaves, stems, bulbs, and flowers. Because most vegetables include water and fiber, they may be consumed in big amounts. A good source of potassium, they are chock-full of nutrients. It's a mineral that's in the proper amount. Sodium is a key player in the body's control of blood pressure. Potassium supplementation is just as critical for those with hypertension as cutting down on salt consumption.

Green leafy veggies are one of the best sources of nutrients. They are rich in minerals, vitamins, and chlorophyll, all of which help to cleanse the body, particularly the liver, including vitamins K, A, C, and folic acid. Vegetables may be used to cocktails or fruit soups if you're sick of salads. The amount of pureed vegetables is greatly reduced. You'll find a variety of lettuces and other vegetables, as well as meat in this dish. Tats and salt grass are among the many ingredients that make up Chinese cabbage.

Compound carbohydrates and starch are often found in root cultures. In order to break down the starch particles more readily, they are frequently cooked before consuming. However, in North

America, raw carrots and radishes are common-place. There are a wide variety of tubers, such as carrots, beets and parsnips. Beets, radishes, and turnips, for example, all have leaves on them. delicious

Sources of inflammation of this group are onions, leeks and garlic. Strengthening the reputation, garlic affects the cardiovascular system. Several studies have shown that it lowers cholesterol, prevents platelet aggregation (when platelets clump together to form blood clots), and lowers blood pressure. Onions are also recommended. Cardiovascular antioniterveyteen because they contain sulfur compounds that garlic is very strong.stalksStem vegetables include asparagus, celery and cabbage. These green vegetables are very nutritious and contain very few calories. Cabbage is a relative of cabbage and broccoli, so it has a strong anti-inflammatory and anti-cancer connection in the cruciferous family. live gameAlthough some of these vegetables are useful in terms of nutrition and cooking, they fall under the category of vegetables. These vegetables have a high water content and shrink significantly when cooked. Because of the variety of vegetables in this class, their nutritional profile is quite diverse, but grapes are high in carotenoids and vitamin C. Vines include squash, pumpkin, eggplant, cucumbers, peas, leaves, tomatoes and peppers. flowerYes, flowers can be vegetables too! This group includes broccoli, cauliflower and artichokes. Broccoli, like most dark green vegetables, is packed with nutrients and antioxidants. Cauliflower is colorless, has similar nutrients and is better for you than broccolimushroomMushrooms are not actually plants (they are fungi), but they are nutritionally similar to vegetables. The difference between fungi is that they eat organic matter and do not use photosynthesis like plants because they are completely different organisms than other vegetables. They are valuable in our diet because they provide various nutrients such as selenium and copper, as well as powerful anti-inflammatory compounds that protect against heart disease, cancer and protect and support the immune system. Mushrooms are rich in minerals and protein calories and are a good source of B vitamins. Some of the mushrooms that can be found in the local market are chandelier, shiitake, oyster, worm, button, nest, and mushroom. There are many edible mushrooms that are used in Chinese medicine for their medicinal properties. Some of them are strong enough to fight cancer.fruitsLike vegetables, fruits are rich in water and fiber, as well as vitamins and minerals. Fruits are an excellent source of quick energy because they are the fastest broken down and used by the body of all the food groups. Fruits contain powerful antioxidants and, because they are sweet, often taste better than vegetables, especially for children. Tree fruit is available in summer and fall, including apples, pears, plums and peaches. Citrus fruits are best in winter, including oranges, grapefruits, lemons and limes. Pure citrus juice can be used to flavor many vegetarian dishes, including vegetables. Summer fruits are berries, grapes and melons. Tropical fruits include banana, pineapple, mango and kiwi.Nuts and seedsNuts and seeds are an excellent source of powerful nutrients, especially minerals and healthy fats, which help the body absorb and fully utilize these minerals. Studies show that people who eat nuts have a lower risk of heart disease. Nuts are good to eat, there are many different types of nuts and seeds because they all have different nutrients. Almonds, walnuts, pistachios, cashews, walnuts, pumpkin seeds, sesame and flax seeds are common.vegetablesBeans Legumes; We usually eat fruits or seeds. They are an excellent source of the amino acid lysine, fiber, vitamins and minerals and are low in fat. They contain healthier proteins than animal products and are also cheaper per gram of protein. Peas, beans, lentils, peanuts and alfalfa are well-known vegetables.Whole grainWhole grains contain complex carbohydrates for energy and are a source of fiber, protein, vitamins (especially vitamins B, A and E), minerals, fatty acids and antioxidants. They are very difficult to digest, so they are usually boiled. outer shells while others have a shell with a soft seed inside. Instead of white, refined or refined grains that contain only starch cells, always choose whole grains with all the nutrients.

Today, a wide variety of whole grains are available in a variety of textures and flavors. N ä is rice, millet, buckwheat, oats, quinoa, spelt, barley and amaranth.Spices and herbsSpices and herbs are not only a way to add rich flavor to dishes, they also contain small amounts of important nutrients. A study of Indian vegetarians showed that they get 39-79% of essential Spices include amino acids, roughly 6% calcium, and 4% iron. There are a lot of sophisticated goods out there that don't have these essential aspects of the diet. White rice, white flour, white sugar, and refined oils like rapeseed are all examples of products that have undergone this process. Fiber, protein, vitamins, and minerals are lost when food is processed. Starch remains as the major component of the grain after washing, along with trace levels of a variety of nutrients. Because of this, they are referred to as "empty calories" They keep your body supplied with the nutrients it needs, but they add calories to your daily calorie intake.

Invest on healthy foods instead than processed ones.

Everything is made to seem as natural as possible. People should have a diet rich in fresh vegetables, fruit; grain products; legumes; nuts and seeds; as well as lean meats. All of the vitamins, minerals, and antioxidants in these foods are more concentrated if you eat them all. Fiber and water-rich foods fill you full without adding calories, making them ideal for dieters.

The meal should be chewed thoroughly.

In addition to slowing down the pace of a nice meal and making it simpler to tell when you're full, it's also the first stage in the digestive process.

Gas and indigestion may occur if carbs are not chewed well enough.

Avoid overdosing on the medication.

The food served at restaurants is usually far more than you need to consume (unless you are in the eye of a stylish restaurant). Try the recipes and meals in this book to get in touch with the proper areas of your body. The quantity of servings is specified in the recipes. To test this, split the dishes and consume a normal-sized portion of each one. Slow down and learn to regulate your appetite and fullness by chewing carefully. This is the greatest method for determining how much food you should consume, but be careful not to overdo it.

Hey, eat!

The vast majority of diet plans and recipes are devoid of flavor. Take a break from the daily grind and enjoy a lighthearted lunch. It's possible that he's still alive. In this book, you'll find recipes for pizza and veggie hamburgers, as well as burritos, tacos, and fajita-style Mexican fare.

Make sure you take vitamins and other substances

Supplementing with herbal Vitamin B 12 tablets is critical for everyone over 50, even those with digestive issues and those on any kind of diet. It is important to keep in mind that animals do not create vitamin B 12; rather, it is produced by bacteria in the digestive tracts of animals when they digest their food. Supplements are the best option for elderly and ruoansulatushäiriöiset persons who are unable to get B12 through diet.

Vitamin B12's RDA in the United States is 24 micrograms per day for most individuals and 28 micrograms per day for pregnant or lactating women, respectively. More recent studies have shown that a daily optimum output of 4-7 micrograms may be achieved using new techniques. It is preferable to take Vitamins B in the morning and early afternoon so that they do not combine before going to sleep.

Calcium absorption and utilization will be compromised if vitamin D deficiency is present. Bones become brittle when calcium and vitamin D levels are low. Vitamin D deficiency is now being linked to everything from asthma to cancer by researchers. Carnivores, too, need to be aware of this and do their part. A 2009 study found that 59% of vegetarians and 64% of meat eaters lacked adequate vitamin D levels.

Vitamin D is not found in vegetarian foods, but our bodies produce it naturally when we are exposed to the sun. Due to the fact that we produce a wide range of mucous membranes and other factors, such as the lack of sunlight in the winter, it is difficult to measure and count. Winter depletes vitamin D levels the farther north you go, and if you live too far north, you may not get any at all. Even though 600 IU is the recommended daily dose, research shows that supplementing with 1,000-2,000 IU is beneficial for the majority of people. Most adults can safely take up to 4000 IU.

Vitamin D deficiency is not always caused by a lack of calcium in the diet, and vegetable sources are often preferable to dairy products because they contain magnesium, which aids in mineral absorption. Getting enough calcium without consuming excessive calories is difficult because of its importance as a nutrient. The recommended daily intake for adults is 1000 mg, which is 700 mg more than the average daily intake of food (up to 1300 mg for the elderly). An add-on that allows you to increase these 300mg more may be of benefit.

Our body also needs two special fatty acids from our diet: omega-3 and omega-6. Others can occur in our bodies if we usually eat enough fat. The difficulty is that our body needs a certain amount of omega-3 to omega-6 fatty acids. Most dietary sources contain too much omega-6 fatty acids, which results in a relative lack of omega-3 fatty acids. The strongest dietary sources of omega-3 fatty acids are ground flaxseeds, flaxseed oil, chia seeds and sachainchi oil, and amazon oil. The ground flaxseeds are large but can be difficult to digest and absorb. If you want to get enough omega-3 fatty acids, oils Linen, Chia and sachainchi (also known as Inca nuts) are great ways to do this.

There is a special type of omega-3 called DHA that is important for brain and nerve function. Your body converts omega-3 to DHA, but it's not always effective. Taking DHA 200-300 mg is often the best way to get this nutrient. People who need more long-chain n-3, such as women in pregnancy and breastfeeding, children and people with digestive or nervous problems , benefit from supplementing DHA with plenty.

Digestive enzyme supplements and / or probiotics may be helpful when switching to a vegetarian diet if you have problems digesting beans. Incomplete digestion is one of the major causes of nutritional deficiencies, as well as food allergies and intolerances. They need antibiotics after probiotics to colonize a healthy intestinal flora.

FOODS

To succeed and take responsibility, you need to model the environment according to your goals, starting with what is brought to the kitchen and putting it on your body. If you make sure your kitchen is full of healthy foods, you can always prepare a well-balanced meal. Although you do not have exactly what a particular recipe needs, you will need ingredients that you need to replace. Let's change our kitchen.

Food Storage

We add flour, sugars, and refined oils, and choose healthy, unrefined versions. Serve us with whole grains, beans, legumes and nuts.

• Whole grains (brown rice, quinoa, buckwheat, millet) (brown rice, quinoa, buckwheat, millet).

• Beans and legumes (chick peas, beans, lentils) (chick peas, beans, lentils).

• Nuts (raisins, dates, dried apricots, berries) (raisins, dates, dried apricots, berries).

• crude oils (olives, coconuts, roasted sesame seeds) (olives, coconuts, roasted sesame seeds)

• Vinegar (apple, balsamic, wine) (apple, balsamic, wine).

• Wholemeal flour (whole grains, spelled, oats, buckwheat) (whole grains, spelled, oats, buckwheat).

• Unsweetened sweeteners (raw cane sugar such as succinate, coconut sugar, maple syrup, molasses, pure stevia) (raw cane sugar such as succinate, coconut sugar, maple syrup, molasses, pure stevia).

• sea salt.

• Spices (ginger, cumin, coriander, turmeric, pepper, cinnamon) (ginger, cumin, coriander, turmeric, pepper, cinnamon).

• Dried herbs (basil, oregano, thyme, dill, mixed herbs) (basil, oregano, thyme, dill, mixed herbs).

• yeast. \sfridge

We put meat, cheese, milk, eggs and packaged food. We supply fresh products, nuts and seeds and other dairy products.

• Green leaves (lettuce, cabbage, Swiss mainland, spinach) (lettuce, cabbage, Swiss mainland, spinach).

• Fresh herbs and spices (parsley, basil, mint, garlic, ginger) (parsley, basil, mint, garlic, ginger).

• Green / starchy vegetables (cucumber, pepper, green beans, broccoli, mushrooms) (cucumber, pepper, green beans, broccoli, mushrooms).

• Starchy vegetables (carrots, beets, sweet potatoes, winter pumpkin) (carrots, beets, sweet potatoes, winter pumpkin)

• Onions (sweet, red, yellow, green) (sweet, red, yellow, green).

• Fruits (apples, oranges, plums, grapes, melons) (apples, oranges, plums, grapes, melons).

• Nuts and seeds (almonds, nuts, sunflower seeds, chia seeds, flax seeds) (almonds, nuts, sunflower seeds, chia seeds, flax seeds).

• Peanut Butter and Seeds (Peanuts, Almonds, Fish Nuts, Sunflower) (Peanuts, Almonds, Fish Nuts, Sunflower)

• Non-milk milk (almonds, soybeans) (almonds, soybeans).

freezer

Time to get rid of TV dinners, potatoes, frozen waffles, ice cream, cakes and frozen desserts. Store fresh frozen and homemade products.

• Frozen berries, mangoes, melon.

• Ripe frozen banana smoothies and cream sorbets.

• Edamame beans, peas, sweet corn, broccoli, spinach and other frozen whole vegetables.

• Highly cooked and frozen in individual batches (soups, stews, peppers, tomato sauce, vegetable burgers) (soups, stews, peppers, tomato sauce, vegetable burgers)

• Healthy confectionery (cakes, cups, pies, fruit cakes) (cakes, cups, pies, fruit cakes).

Home fast food factory

Sometimes we don't have time to follow the rules. I have now created a draft of a balanced aterista, so you can connect it to the kitchen.

mixer

Prepare a perfect nutritious cocktail to start the day and feed it. You will need:

• Glass and straw: Reusable straws minimize contact with your teeth for better dental health, and the use of an insulated cup or travel mug makes a cocktail known in the morning.

• Creamy: bananas (frozen computer brands such as ice cream), avocados, peanut butter or milk without milk.

• Omega-3: 1 tablespoon of flax or chia seeds.

Protein: a handful of oatmeal or quinoa or a tablespoon of vegetable protein powder.

• Fruit: about 1 cup blueberry, watermelon, grapes, apples L paths of any shape.

• Fortify vegetables: vegetables such as spinach, sprouts or cabbage; vegetables such as cucumbers or carrots; Fresh herbs such as mint or basil.

• Rise of food baskets: fresh ginger, powdered green leaves, matcha powder, probiotics, berries or goji powder, cocoa beans.

bowl

Build the perfect bowl for lunch or dinner that will provide you with all the nutrients and fuel you need for the rest of the day. You will need:

Bowl: Get a pair of the same size to hold the same portions

• Green leafy vegetables: Take a handful or two as much as you want, lettuce, cheeseburger, spinach, cabbage, Swiss lime, parsley or other vegetables.

• Starchy vegetables and / or whole grains: About 1 cup sweet potatoes, winter pumpkin, brown rice, quinoa, spelled, Soba noodles, rice noodles, etc.

• Beans or legumes: about ½ cup beans, black beans, lentils, edamame or other legumes.

• Other vegetables: about 1 cup of raw vegetables such as cucumber, pepper, tomato and avoca-

do; grilled such as zucchini, eggplant and mushrooms; or steamed like broccoli, carrot and beetroot.

Peanut butter or a small handful of nuts (pumpkin, cashew, almond) may serve as a sauce basis.

Long and luscious fillet of sauce. Test out some
of the recipes in this book, including the sesame
and baked misokastiketta, the jumalatarikastiket-
ta green, or the creamy balsamikastiketta, or go
through the ingredients to make your own.

Groups of foods

In terms of heart health, herbal diets are
well-known for their importance to our overall
well-being and health. Researchers, on the other
hand, say that certain herbal diets may be dam-
aging to health, as Fred's father learned the hard
way. Your heart's health is at stake here.

The CDC estimates that 600,000 Americans die each year as a result of cardiovascular disease. Poor diet, a major contributor to heart disease, has been blamed for this fatality.

In the last several decades, many studies have shown the health advantages of a diet rich in whole grains and other plant-based foods including legumes, flaxseeds, and fruits.

Vegetables were shown to be the greatest kind of food for people and their health, according to another study.

Herbal diets include both advantages and drawbacks, according to the most recent thorough research. About 209,289 people participated in the research, according to the nurses and medical experts who performed it. It took the researchers roughly two decades to learn about the daily habits, health habits, and medical histories of the individuals. They have never had a stroke, cancer or cardiac surgery in their lives. About 8,631 coronary artery disease patients were surveyed for follow-up.

There is a big difference between vegetarian and vegetarian diets, which is why these studies are so important. On the basis of advantages and disadvantages, he wanted to categorize vegetarians.

Diets were the primary focus of the study, and three distinct diets were created by the researchers:

Vegetarian diet based on harmful plant foods. Refined cereals, sugary drinks, candies, and potatoes are among them.

Diets that permit the consumption of animal products and nutrients while yet adhering to the dietary restrictions of vegetarians.

Plant-based herbal products with an emphasis on entire grains, vegetables, fruit, and legumes (these products are more organic).

Chapter Four

A GUIDE TO FOOD DESIGN BUILDINGS

The best thing you can do is to buy fresh produce

Wherever feasible, buy locally sourced and organically grown items whenever possible. Expand yours if you can. On a windowsill, you may easily cultivate sprouts and herbs. Replace the old jyvi s and spices in your cupboard after approximately a year if you use them all. A better-tasting dinner is a given when you start with high-quality components.

The things you wish to buy are at your fingertips.

You should eat a lot of veggies and other high-quality foods. Introducing new members to the group is a good way to keep things fresh, but it's not always the case. For the vast majority of individuals, certain foods are more palatable than others. They're more appealing because of their inherent sweetness, which comes from things like pumpkins and sweet potatoes. Freshly picked or young plants have a more delicate flavor and texture than their mature counterparts.

Cooking techniques may be chosen.

Use the proper manner of cooking. Avocados, broccoli, and sweet potatoes and squash may all be cooked in the oven or on the stovetop to great effect. A variety of cooking methods may be used to enhance the taste of whole grains, including pre-cooking.

Select the best possible combinations.

Aromas (sweet, salty, and sour) and textures combine in this dish's meal combo (crisp, sweet). In addition to the vase's aesthetic attractiveness, color has a significant impact on its visual appeal. He's looking for a way to bring together opposites (bitter) or similarities (similarity) (all greens). Since these are only preferences, you should experiment with the data in the recipes and see what you think.

Add salt to the solution.

A modest quantity of salt may have a significant impact on the flavor and texture of food, especially vegetables, by lowering their bitterness and increasing their fluidity. As a result, plant cells melt more easily from the inside out as a result of this treatment. Hummus may be made using a wide variety of components, so it doesn't know what each one is. When preparing food, season it with salt, massage it into the veggies to moisten them, or drizzle a little salted sauce over the dish or salad.

Beans should be seasoned.

Beans and other legumes aren't very appetizing. Improve their appeal by: • Adding healthy, mouthwatering fruits or vegetables to the mix.

While the water is coming to a boil, seasonings such as herbs and spices may be added.

Spices and salty sauces may be used to enhance the flavor of the vegetable broth or juice.

cordially

Spices and sauces may enhance the flavor of any food. The harshness and texture of the vegetables are softened and the flavors of the veggies and sauce are combined when they are cooked with chopped vegetables in a nice sauce. For an hour or more, marinate the beans and all of the beans in the sauce so that they are infused with the sauce's flavor.

Add a piece of cake or a piece of

In the kitchen, use natural sweeteners. Salads and soups benefit from the addition of fruits such as apples, oranges, dried cranberries, and raisins.

Make use of heart-healthy lipids.

Fat enhances the flavor and texture of a meal. For those of us who like our food hot and spicy in the evening and yrtteiltä, fats are the way to go. A few days later, or if you aren't used to healthful cooking, you may feel the effects of a high-carbo-hydrate, low-fat vegetarian diet. Exercise and eat foods high in fats like nuts, seeds, and avocados instead of boiling meals that naturally contain fat.

The cream basis for a sauce or sauce is a blend of peanut butter and seeds or avocado.

camouflage

Consider the consequences of your actions. Make soups, sauces, or drinks by combining vegetables and vegetables. Carrot cake, zucchini bread, pumpkin muffins, chocolate beetroot infusion, and sweet potato cakes are just some of the veggie delicacies you may bake.

Planned events

To what extent will your food's nutritional, taste, and energy content be enhanced? Everything is possible right now, I can guarantee you that! My goal with these meal plans is to teach you how to cook tasty herbal meals that give a well-balanced diet and nutrients.

The kitchen's veggie diet will be free of assumptions for the next three weeks. In a matter of weeks, there are three meals a day plus snack alternatives available. More recipes than meal plans may be found in Chapter 3. As a result, you have some leeway if one of your meal plans isn't working well for you.

Because most of us do not have the time to cook three meals a day, these meal plans make use of leftovers. Monday through Friday, students are expected to bring and pick up their own breakfast and lunch. My advise includes how to plan for the week so that you may be ready for success.

Chapter 11 sweets aren't included in the plan, but if you'd want to bring something sweet to a party or a dinner, you're free to do so.

It's important for us to finish this plan feeling good about ourselves, so we've set some goals to help us achieve that aim.

Take a few snoozes

Sleep has been shown to have an effect on the portion of the brain that governs one's ability to resist temptation. As a result, it is more difficult to resist temptation if you are awake. The inability to make clear judgments raises the probability that he may consume something he doesn't intend to eat.

Because it cannot handle stress in a productive manner, it is more likely to overeat or engage in other harmful compensatory behaviors. In addition to making you healthier and more energized, regular, high-quality sleep helps you control your urges. A good night's sleep may be achieved in a number of ways.

• Keep your sleep and wake-up times consistent each day.

30 minutes before going to bed, turn off all electronic devices (TV, computer, tablet, phone).

• Don't work out after eating a meal.

after 2 pM, caffeine deficit becomes apparent

• No sugar after lunch.

The night before you go to bed, try a calming activity like restorative yoga or meditation.

Three times a week, I'm active.

Getting regular exercise is important for a healthy heart, strong bones, a healthy lymphatic system, and a strong immune system. It may also assist to avoid diabetes. Exercising releases hormones into the bloodstream that make you feel good, decrease your desire for food, and generally keep your body in good working order. A fast exercise after work may make it less appealing as a supper option.

Regular physical activity may improve your mood and your capacity to deal with stressful circumstances by reducing weariness, sadness, tension, anxiety, and discomfort. Your body will run more effectively as you gain strength and resistance. If you want to walk or roller skate or hula hula, start there. If you like something, you're more likely to continue to enjoy it in the long run. semester. Three times a week, demonstrate a skill that you can do for 20-30 minutes. In order to keep you interested, it doesn't always have to be the same blend. Once you have the hang of it, you may add more days, spend more time, or attempt something more extreme.

Don't put too much emphasis on being flawless.

Stress has a negative impact on health, and severe food stress is detrimental. For the most part, I don't know anybody who can keep an excellent nutrition plan while also exercising every day. If you have a bad day, you'll feel bad about it since it will only bring you bad energy. It's common for individuals to overeat while they're sick. To avoid using terms like "slip," "trap," or "bug," I've chosen not to. Everything we do is a part of who we are and helps us become the person we want to be. I already know what day it is going to be tomorrow

Do not punish yourself by reducing your calorie intake or increasing your physical activity. Make your intentions for the future work for you in the present by writing a letter every day.

Pay attention to your body's signals and have fun with it!

Finding the appropriate balance for your body's demands does not necessarily need following a rigid diet or rulebook. With a renewed interest in your health, you may reconnect with your intuition and use it to discover what works best for you.Eat consciously, chew food well, taste and taste when you eat enough

With your body in balance and following the principles of a long-term healthy diet, you should be able to hear your body's messages about what should be healthy. Every person is different and has a different way of being healthy. However, your body's messages can be distorted or muted when they are unbalanced, so it is difficult to determine at first whether you think there is real desire or hunger.

Positive energy can have a big impact on your goals. It is unfortunate that many diet programs focus on avoiding unhealthy foods by switching to a healthy diet because it is much nicer and more effective to focus on eating good foods. such as fruits, nuts, or a special dinner, and eat them often to keep you happy and excited about a healthy lifestyle.

Chapter Five

WEEKU VEGAN'S MANUFACTURING PLAN

week

CONTRACT NOTICE

Breakfast: vanilla, pudding 1 tablespoon fresh soda

Lunh: Fluffy Crisp and Open Water Low in Oil or Sweet Potato (Marinated)

Snorkel behind: 1/4 cups hemp powder with fresh vegetables (wrinkles, flowers, romaine salad, balls, etc.)

Dinner: Black beans and salad uinoa salad q uick cumin drosesing

DESSERT: Spider shock

Tuesday

Winds are as follows: Cocktail, 1 almond raisin, 1 tear, banana, 1, 2 times.

Lunch: 1 brown roasted coffee (for toast) or two gluten-free cakes with fresh or toasted 1/4 hummus tortilla are a bit strong. SEE FLOWERING EQUIPMENT WELCOME OR DURING.

After a snack: a protein bar

Lunch: Zuchini pasta with chryrry tomatoes, sweet potatoes, balsam and hemp.

DESSERT: BANANA SUPPORT

Wednesday

Best for: Fifth success as soon as possible with 1 tbsp fresh beans

Food: said at least three cups of green vegetables you would like to get 3 caps or treasures and one from Koszenocero.

Afternoon snack: 4 tablespoons of hummingbird with fresh vegetables (wrinkles, celery, lettuce, balls, etc.)

Dinner: Cappuccino,

Dessert: 2 pieces of raw brownies

Thursday

Best for: Nirvana chillies and chocolate, fresh fruit is recommended

LUNH: I just made a salad with 1/2 cup of organic drink

Behind the snorkel: 1 ounce. Almonds and a few tablespoons of raisins

Lunch: Summer quiz and perfect spot (obtained from q or uinnaa paacta for brown)

PROJECT: 2 EXTREMELY EXCLUSIVE MASSAGES

Friday

More importantly, a smiling face with 1 cup of almonds, 1 cup of berries, 1 cup of nutritious chocolate chocolate, 3 tablespoons of salads and 1 cup of coffee milk.

€ 15.00

Snout: 2 options with almond butter

Dinner: Buttruther s ash curry serves the way cup cooked q uinoa, steamedeeeeтables as desire d

Dessert: dark chocolates

Saturday

Breakfast: oatmeal and almond butter

Lunh: Smiley, avoid and say jícam

Snack back: 1 tablespoon of almonds mixed with nutritional protein powder and several cubes

DENNER: Burgers and Black Grains, Served with Small Salad or Steamed Vegetables

Dessert: 2 types of vanilla and vanilla

Sundays

Breakfast: small 1/2 ice cream, 1 cup ice, 2 ice cubes, 3/4 cups starch, 1 cup green leafy vegetables and 1 serving of nutritious vanilla.

Lunh: He left the previous burger and burger, he said.

Second snack: 1/4 cup vegan mix (or 2 table-spoons almond or pine nuts and 2 tablespoons dried fruit)

Dinner 1 cup of selected q uinoa, browned rice, or in the case of served Half chopped avocado 1 cup steamede greens and of chomo sauce.

Dessert: 1/2 cup chocolate

ALL WEEKS

On Monday,

Best for: gluten-free banana pancake, served with 1 cup of fresh beans

Lunch: Mango, Kale, and avassal d

Snack: Afternoon, bread, paddle, berrée or other selected fresh fruit.

DENNER: ROLLANTINATION OF EGG VEG-
ETABLES EXAMPLES OF TRUCKS, GOODS
OR BROKOLO

PROJECTS: DARKL SHOCK

Tuesday

Best for: Cinnamon

Lunch: pumpkin and apple soup, served with fresh green vegetables or selected carved vegetables

Afternoon snack: nutrition at the bar

Note: Raw zucchini is eaten with basil and various cakes, served with sauces or such stressful sausages.

PROJECT: 2 vegan cookies

Wednesday

Small addition: Cocktail 1 cut into bluish designs or blends containing 1 cup coconut and half water to be included in plan 1 chocolate according to cooking plan

Lunch: Easy to grow yellow lentil with avocado croutons

Snack: fresh vegetables, 1/4 cup hummus

Day: salad or black rice and amaranth with delicate cumin

DESIGN: 1/2 cups from the collection

Thursday

Most important: 1 bread bath, 1 cup of organic or delicious coffee (I like white bread) and 1 cup of almond milk

Lunch: apples, portions and crispy curry sauce

Previous answer: 1/4 cups of real powder mixture according to your choice

Dinner: SWETT POTATATE LIMMER BURBERERS, say first or say VEGETAL as he wanted

DESIGN: 2 raw vanilla noodles

Friday

Best: VANILLA butter pudding with 1 cup fresh soda

Lunch: The front, is outside, and said many rockets.

Afternoon: Group of walnuts and raw walnut jelly

Lunch: sweet potatoes and milk are made with broccoli or steamed vegetables

PROJECT: 1/2 Chocolate

WEEKU VEGAN'S MANUFACTURING PLAN

Saturday

Breakfast: Smoothie with 1 frozen banana, 1/2 tablespoon fried mango, 1 tablespoon hippie, 1 cup avocado and 1/2 cup coconut.

Lunch: WHITE LOOP LORD AND USE CHILD OR GREEN GREEN

Afternoon snack: Nutrition instead of choice

Lunch: "Rice" with lemon, lemon and pistachios, served with fresh vegetables

PROJECT: DELIVERY OF RAW MILK

Sunday

Best: BANANA AND FEES

Lunch: An avocado carrot is a good buy for a salad.

Snorkel Back: Raw vegetables with sweet potato humus

Lunch: brown rice with lentils, served with fresh salad or steamed vegetables and for eating.

Dessert: 2 many misc

CONTINUE THREE

CONTRACT NOTICE

Best for: gia with stiff pudding with chia

Lunch: leftover brown rice and lentils, lots of mixed vegetables and many reception options.

Afternoon aperitif: 2 scoops of peanut butter and snacks

Note: Raw "nuts" are not consumed with steamed vegetables or at your discretion.

DESIGN: Dark chocolate

Teseas

Breakfast: cocktail with 1 glass of almonds, 1 large frozen bread, 1-2 tablespoons at a time, 1 serving of powder and cup filled with granules, lots and lots of grains.

Lunch: mango, avocado and avocado

Afternoon Snack: True Vegetarian and HUM-MUS ANNUAL REPORT

Lunch: Easy rice without beans and vegetables

Dessert: 2 raw and vegan cookies

Wednesday

Breakfast: BANANAN BRAAKFASS WRAPS

Lunh: Omelette and fresh fish salad.

Snack: Restaurant Bar

Lunch: Arugulana with cooking and fruits, blue-berries and tasty

PROJECT: Banana contains something else

Thursday

Best for: Cinnamon Apple

Lunch: fennel salad, avocado and tomatoes 1/2 tbsp white beans or white beans

Snack: 1 group of people mixed with protective powder

Lunch: It is said that most baked cakes are tinned.

Dessert: dark chocolates

Friday

Breakfast: gluten-free vegan muffins with a spoon of almond butter and a plate

Lunch: apples, portions and chrysanthemum; 1 cup rice and mushroom soup

Snack: 1/3 cup raw fruit mix (or a mix of almonds, raisins or jelly beans)

Lunch: some mustard is cut into large pieces and "weeping" and "weeping" steamed with boiled broccoli or broccoli.

PROJECT: Waffle ginger is creamy

Saturday

In a nutshell: SmOththie with 1 ½ cups of blue water or fruit mixture, 1 grape with nuts, 1/2 small amount of water, 1 high surface resistance.

Lunh: easily wrapped in "croutons", served with lots of sauces or steamed drinks.

After a snack: Officer sticks stored 2 tablespoons of nuts or almonds and raisins ("ants in logs")

Note: After a large amount of raw vegetables and selected vegetables, 1 cup cooked oysters, 1/2 ½ cup, ½ cup, ½ cup of coffee, ingredients and unique label sauce.

PROJECT: 2 rare, highly visible

Sunday

Key Features: 1 slice of banana and fresh fruit, rice, 1 cup or organic millet, full of rice (I like the Arrowhead Mills brand) and 1 cup of corn.

Lunch: smoked avocado and jicama, 1 small, if desired

Back snorkel: 2 balls of walnuts and Japanese cereal straight

Dinner: Quinnaencillas

Dessert: Sugar chocolate

Four weeks

CONTRACT NOTICE

Most importantly, cut 1 frozen banana, 1/2 frozen Mug, 1 canola, 1 tablespoon coconut and 1/2 cup wine

Lunch: leftover food in the kitchen, talking to selected salad dressing

Snack: Selected food bar

Lunch: Arugulá declared the roasted pumpkin, swallowed it, and fled.

PROJECT: 2 EXTREMELY EXCLUSIVE MAS-SAGES

Tuesday

Breakfast: Vánnila can hug one cup of fresh berries

Dinner: the red flame and finally the ragula said in good taste

Afternoon snack: lots of raw peanut butter and jelly beans

Dinner: The offer of sweets and black beans is made from broccoli or coarse.

Dessert: 1/2 cup chocolate

Wednesday

Best for: 1 cocktail of frozen bread, 1/2 table-spoon of frozen ice cream, 1 tablespoon of spinach leaves, 1 cup of avocado nuts and 1/2 cup of wine

Lunh: Boll with smaller black beans and sweet potatoes in large quantities.

Next dive: diet choice

Lunch: Cauliflower "water" with lemon, mint and beans stored in large quantities

Dessert: Serve chocolate with almonds

Thursday

Note: Smiling face with 1 tablespoon of almonds, 1 large frozen banana, 1-2 tablespoons at a time, 1 serving of protein powder and lots of creams (spinach, approx.

Lunch: 1 freshly made rice tortilla (for life) or oatmeal with 1/4 inch cocoa tortillas, roasted or roasted peppers and lots of green leaves. Serve if desired with steamed vegetables or in a small dish.

Diving Back: Basic Nutrition

DENNER: zucchini paste with tomato cake, sweet potato, basil and parmesan cheese

Dessert: soft banana

Friday

Most important: Apple introduces itself right away

Lunch: fried pumpkin and big soup, served with steamed or steamed vegetables

Afternoon snack: nutrition bar

DENNER: Raw ZuChin with Alfredo cherry and cherry tomato, served with fresh salads or vegetables of your choice.

PROJECT: 2 real brownie rats

Saturday

Best of all: smiling face 1 cup frozen or mixed berries, 1 cup walnut water, 1/2 small avocado, 1 serving chocolate and a pinch of porridge.

Lunch: Easy avocado curry with lentils

Afternoon snack: fresh vegetable greens, 1/4-caries

Denner: BANK granular and nos uinoina talked about dressing uikkum Cuminn Dressing

DESIGN: 1/2 cups from the collection

Sundays

The most important thing: VANILLA can pudding with 1 tablespoon of fresh beans

Lunh: Crisp red and green, looks like a little 1 tbsp sweet potatoes (or 1 small potato, packaged)

Afternoon snack: 1/4 cup hummingbird with fresh vegetables (horns, frogs, romantic leaves, balls, etc.)

FOOD : UNO INOALA BANK AND SALAD IN A FAST COMMUNITY PROJECT

Chapter Six

STARTING UP PLANET BASE

Statistics show that more and more people are choosing a plant-based diet. People know about the benefits of a plant-based diet. In the United States, one-third of consumers are actively consuming more plant-based foods. Celebrities such as Formula 1 champion Lewis Hamilton, I'm Will, award-winning Hollywood director Ava DuVernay, screenwriter Alicia Silverstone, actress and musician Moby have also supported the herb. Why use a plant-based diet? According to various studies and research, a plant-based diet is known to prevent and reverse type 2 diabetes and advanced cardiovascular disease.Research also shows that people who follow a plant-based diet can lose weight more easily and reduce their risk of sudden death and heart disease. Doctors, nutritionists and health experts have constantly used a plant diet to treat and prevent cholesterol (and evil), hypertension and certain types of c ancer.In Las Vegas, it is a rocky spirit of ELN (including food, growth alcohol, vegetables), with a healthy diet, regardless of childhood, teens, young, pregnancy and aging. For all foods, regard- less of age and best for everyone, athletes can choose this diet. I'm sure the profits will suffer. I pointed it out and was happy to get on the train. Despite the importance of these points, you should understand that change is somewhat diffi- cult. Some wanted to leave, but could not prove it.This means that your primordial energy must be strong enough to support you in this lifestyle. It involves a lot of planning, determination and commitment.I had to ask my clients to move little by little. If you've been drinking soda and popcorn every day for the past 10 years, it's nearly impossible to go a week without them.Here are some simple techniques that have helped me and my clients get through herbal and water solutions. Start with small stepsSwitching to a plant-based diet is no different than spending months learning to walk on one leg. It is best to start with a simple vegetarian diet. This could be a bean and rice burrito, oatmeal, three roasted peppers, spaghetti spring rolls, roasted vegetables or le ntils.Thus, you can start preparing these dishes step by step. Choosing such food is a good way, because only human nature is devoted to our love. Better to build slowly because it takes the pressure off you know in the beginning. Reduce your consumption of processed foods and meat. Instead of cutting out meat and processed foods, you can also reduce your consumption of animal products and processed foods. Change the ratio to 80:20, 70:30, 60:40, 50:50, 45:55, 40:60, 30:70, 20:80, 10:90 to get 100% vegetarian food. The first set of numbers refers to processed foods, meat and animal products, while the second set refers to plant-based foods. By doing this, you give your mind and body time to adjust to this diet. To begin with, you can add a few table-spoons of salad to your diet, and then replace the meat with vegetable alternatives such as porto-bello or dried Bulgarian mushrooms. Start with a healthy vegetarian breakfastAfter the first two steps, you can proceed to the third - a daily vegetable breakfast. Make it your first meal to gradually warm up your body. Once balanced, go to lunch and then adjust your snacks and dinnerCheck your protein intakeAlthough our bodies need one gram of protein per kilogram of body weight, many people get enough each day.The body's need for protein is not a reason to consume too much of it, as it can be harmful to the body. You just need to find a food that can provide you with the 9 essential amino acids that your body really needs.It is good that healthy plant food contains proteins and amino acids in different proportions. It's easy to focus on whole foods, as long as you're getting the right amount of calories your body needs. It also means that the protein deficiency is severe. You know what you spend onYou must know what you are doing and how to prepare proper and healthy food for yourself. There are many plant-based products on the market, such as cheese and curd, but they are very complex. It is very bad for the body because it is very saturated with saturated fat, amino acids, flour, salt, refined oil and sugar.So it's best to know what you're buying and read the label before you buy. Research and choose organic and whole foods. try ä read the nutrition and breeding s mit s sy o t. L ö will find s variety of ways to prepare various dishes.

If you can, hire a vegetarian dietitian to help her plan and choose the best meals. I was able to do this for people, which made the transition easier for my clients. This lifestyle can be difficult, but with the help of a nutritionist, it's easy.He althy eating never stopsThere are many healthy foods that you can easily find by visiting supermarkets and convenience stores. This makes it easy to integrate herbal products and lifestyles. Contains dairy-free milk, tofu, potato and tempeh. Regardless of the price, the next time you go to the supermarket, you can look at the vegan and fresh products. There is never a shortage of healthy and nutritious food. Keep a few in your bag, drawers, work area, fridge and workshop. Be creative with what you eatStart eating and learn how creativity works. You can learn to cook and try something new for yourself. The more you try, the better you get. Discover new ways to prepare salads, soups and daily meals so you don't waste time eating the same food every day.Eat snacks whenever you want (I'll show you how to make them in the next sections). Take the time to learn recipes from various blogs and restaurants.Find a groupSocial media makes it easy to connect with anyone or anything. Find groups to help you learn and learn new skills. They can cheer you up when you need it and teach you what to do when your cravings hit. You can also ask questions. All in all, you should look like a toddler learning. That way you won't force yourself to study. Find one that works for you and stick with it.Creating building services of 50 important food principlesWe talked for a long time about what to eat and when to work. Now you have to know how to do what is good for you. This is the only way to be 100% sure of what you are eating. I teach you how to cook all plant-based meals and what to do with vegetables, fruits, legumes, tubers, grains and other whole foods. I give you recipes of all kinds of food from all over the world. It doesn't matter if you are a novice or a chef. I am sure you will learn something new or improve yourself. I am sure that one day you will create miracles in your kitchen. receiptWe use and enjoy the information in the recipes. In the following chapters, I will give you more than 100 recipes that will help you discover the flavors of vegetarianism, and I hope you will enjoy this lifestyle. These recipes have high fat, saturated fat, balanced sodium and potassium, healthy heart and antioxidants. All of them have immunity and anti -inflammatory properties, due to some specific materials that indicate what instructions for children without nuts, no herbs and a fast product (15 minutes or less, appropriate, some of the recipes are appropriate. I will mention turbochargers in this area.). In addition to the meal plan, there are many delicious and nutritious meals and desserts, so you can enjoy healthy meals for a long time.M aximum vibration powerMakes 3-4 cups. Preparation time: 5 minutesA quick gluten-free preparation, which is an anti-inflammatory agent to strengthen immunity, is suitable for childrenIt is a great breakfast base to start the day with extra nutrients to increase nutrient density.Shoots and fires are difficult, so it is better to tear the leaves from the stem and work only with the leaves. Vegetables and carrots work best if you have a high-powered blender, such as a Blendtec or Vit amix.If you have a regular blender, skip the fresh greens and use green powder as a vegetable brand and brittle needles for nutrients. to shakePrepare the required 3 cupsPreparation time: 5 minutes

Gluten Free PREPARATION FOR NEW IN-FLAMMATION

Chai spices can help digestion, improve glycemic control and increase metabolism. Chia seeds are a fantastic source of omega-3 fatty acids, calcium, phosphorus and manganese. Prepare these delicious cocktails to enjoy your trip as an alternative to the highly nutritious Lai Chai.

Chapter Seven

THE METHODS

- In a mixer, combine all the ingredients and mix well, adding water as required. • Butter or almond butter • 1 tablespoon maple syrup (optional)

- • 1 cup of alfalfa or chopped spinach (optional)

- A quarter of a cup of fresh, raw milk (optional)

- One cup of water

- SECONDARY LEADERSHIPS (optional)

- 1/4 cup ground maca

- Approximately 1 tbsp.

- 1 Place all ingredients in a blender and process until smooth, adding extra water (or milk) as necessary.

- 2 As required, provide more changes. Mash is perplexed.

- Shake of the Pink Panther

- Prepare the three glasses of your choice.

- 5 minutes of preparation time

- Swiftly confirmation with little opposition to preparation so that you may drive fast without fear.

- Cocktail has a silky feel to it, with nothing in the way of dynamism to it. Many unique nutrients in berries, such as vitamin C, antioxidants, anti-inflammatory, and liver and urinary tract infection prevention, are found in berries. Berries are a significant source of vitamin C.

- In addition, 1 cup of strawberries

- Cut melon into 1 cup serving size pieces (all types)

- One cup of raspberries or blueberries.

- • 1 tbsp. chia seeds

- • 12 cups of coconut milk or alternative milk may be used.

- One cup of water

- SECONDARY LEADERSHIPS (optional)

- Goji berries in a teaspoon

- Fresh cut mint leaves, about 2 teaspoons

- instructions:

- Stir in extra water (or coconut milk) as necessary to get desired smoothness in the blender. 1

- 2 As required, provide more changes. Mash is perplexed.

- 5 minutes of preparation time

- EXCLUSIVELY WITHOUT CHILDREN

- It's like eating a slice of banana bread. Prepare a simple meal or dessert in a jiffy. If you don't have a powerful blender, you may make a wonderful alternative to almond butter that has 2 tablespoons of nuts instead of almond butter. Mußli or Mußli with fresh fruit slices in a bowl

- • 1 banana

- • 1 tbsp. almond or sunflower butter

- cinnamon powder, about 14 teaspoon

- In order to add a little nutmeg flavor:

- 2 Tbsp. Maple Syrup •

- There should be 1 tablespoon of flax or hemp seeds in each of your meals

- A quarter of a cup of fresh, raw milk (optional)

- One cup of water

- Add extra water (or non-milk) if necessary to ensure that the blender is thoroughly cleaned.

-

Cooking time: 5 minutes or overnight / Preparation time: 5 minutes.

- gluten-free cooking without the presence of children's pals

- Heart-healthy oats are a staple in many diets. Beta-glucan fibers, which decrease cholesterol utilizing antioxidants, avantan-tamides, which may help cleanse blood vessel walls, and lignans, which protect against heart disease, are enticing packets." He's basically a super hero in the form of his humble oats.

- • 12 cup gluten-free oatmeal or quinoa

- — 1 tablespoon chia seeds, flax seeds, or hemp seeds crushed

-

This recipe calls for 1 tablespoon maple syrup or coconut sugar (optional)

- • 14 tsp. cinnamon powder (optional)

- AVAILABILITY OF SPECIAL ORDER ITEMS

- Nuts with a quartered apple

- Dry cranberries and pumpkin seeds make a great snack.

- There should be at least one diced pear and at least one tablespoon of cashew butter.

- • 1 cup of grapes, diced, and 1 tablespoon of sunflower seeds

- • 1 diced banana and 1 tablespoon peanut butter

- A serving of raisins and hazelnuts contains 2 teaspoons of each ingredient.

- • 1 cup of blueberries and 1 tablespoon of unsweetened coconut flakes

- If you'd like to skip this step, combine oat flakes with linseed, maple syrup, and cinnamon in a separate dish (travel cup or short thermos works well)

- 2 Soak the oats in cold water, then blend the oats and water. Make sure to soak for at least 30 minutes or longer.

- A region selection option is now included in the new design.

- Oatmeal cookies for breakfast

- Make five large cookies.

- It takes 15 minutes to prepare and 12 minutes to cook.

- Preparation for youngsters may be done in a short time.

- Even if you cook your breakfast in a cookie, it may still be quite nutritious. Think of it as a nutritious bowl of porridge for fun. These cookies are a great way to start the day since they include oatmeal, linseed, almonds, and whole grains, all of which are healthy for cardiovascular health. Sorghum and oats or quinoa may be substituted for conventional porridge to make them gluten-free.

- • 1 tablespoon of ground flax seeds

- Nutella or sunflower butter, 2 tbsp

- For the maple syrup, use 2 teaspoons

- Banana puree, about a tablespoon

- • 1 tsp. cinnamon powder

- • 14 teaspoon nutmeg (optional)

- • A dash of sea salt

- • 12 cup of oats

- Chocolate raisins or shavings in a quarter-cup measure

- Set the oven temperature to 350 degrees Fahrenheit. • 1 Begin by lining a baking sheet with parchment paper and spraying it Spread out a big baking sheet of parchment paper on a counter.

-

Preparation Step 2: Soak the linen in a large bowl with just enough water to cover it and lay it aside

- 3 In a large bowl, combine the almond butter, maple syrup, and banana until smooth. Pour in the linen-and-water concoction combination.

- Add salt and pepper to the wet mixture before adding the cinnamon and nutmeg in a separate bowl.

- 5 Double the oats with raisins.

- 6 Roll the spaghetti into a ball and press it softly into the pan to level the surface. Then repeat the process by spacing the two by 2 to 3 inches from each other.

-

7 To get a golden color, cook for an additional 12 minutes.

- 8 Cookies may be kept in the refrigerator or freezer for later use in an airtight container

- There are two types of flax seeds:

- apple wine vinegar, 1 tsp

- One teaspoon of vanilla extract

- • 12 teaspoon ground cinnamon

- One-half teaspoon of grated, dried ginger (optional)

- • 14 teaspoon nutmeg (optional)

f you'd like, you may add a dash of Jamaican pepper to the mix.

• 12 tsp. baking soda

The Rolling Stones (OPTIONAL)

• 12 cup of oats

• 2 tbsp. raisin or other dried fruit

• 2 teaspoons of sunflower seeds

The oven should be preheated at 350 degrees Fahrenheit. Coconut oil or silicon cups or paper cups may be used to prepare a six-cup muffin pan.

A food processor or pressure cooker may be used for blending all of the ingredients except the vanilla bean and nutmeg.

3 Using a clean coffee grinder, grind the oats into a fine flour (or use whole wheat flour). Mix the oats with baking powder and baking soda in a large bowl.

4 Mix the wet and dry ingredients together until they are completely incorporated. Assemble all of the extras (if you use them)

5 Bake 14 cup of pasta in each loaf for 30 minutes, or until the interior of the rod can be easily pierced with a toothpick. Because of the orange's juicy basis, the rollers may last for up to 30 minutes, depending on the muffin's weight.

A batch of muffins filled with an apple and compote compote is ready to eat.

He creates a total of twelve cups.

Cooking time: 15-20 minutes plus 15 minutes for prepping the ingredients.

Preparation for youngsters may be done in a short time.

They're based on the sandwiches I loved as a kid, but with more veggies and less fat and sugar.

Raw brown sugar such as succinate, date sugar, or other unprocessed powdered sugar may replace coconut sugar, which has a low glycemic index. Adding molasses, nutmeg, demerara, or turbinate that has only been partly refined would be excellent, but brown sugar that is just refined white sugar should be avoided.

When making muffins, use 1 teaspoon of coconut oil to distribute them (optional)

peanut or seed butter, about two teaspoons.

1-1/2 cups unsweetened apple mousse.

• 13 cup of coconut sugar

A quarter of a cup of raw, unpasteurized milk

• 2 tbsp. flax seed powder

apple wine vinegar, 1 tsp

One teaspoon of vanilla extract

• 2 cups of whole grain flour

one-half teaspoon of baking soda

• 12 tsp. baking powder

• 1 rounded teaspoon of cinnamon

• A dash of sea salt

• 12 cup of finely chopped nuts

• Components of the dish (optional)

• 14 cup walnuts

• 1 cup and a quarter of coconut sugar

• 12 teaspoon ground cinnamon

The oven should be preheated at 350 degrees
Fahrenheit. Use coconut oil, silicon cups, or paper cups to line two 6-cup muffin tins and set
aside.

A big bowl should be filled with a mixture of peanut butter and apple mousse as well as coconut sugar, milk, linseed, vinegar, and vanilla.

A third big basin should be filled with flour, baking powder, baking soda, cinnamon and salt.

4 Using your hands, blend the dry and wet ingredients.

5 Fill each muffin two-thirds of the way full with batter, then top with your preferred topping (if using). After 20 to 30 minutes of baking, check to see whether the inside stick of the pan is clean. Because the cans of apple juice produce such a luscious foundation, cupcakes can keep longer.

Bananas with raspberry syrup drenched in buttery, fluffy French bread

A year's worth of Plasterk in bed equals eight.

Cooking time: 30 minutes / Preparation time: 10 minutes.

QUICK PREPARATION FOR FREE KIDS 'FRIENDS

When bananas are substituted for eggs in French toast, a fresh flavor and natural sweetness emerge. Baking isn't necessary. Syrup made from raspberries Because of the richness of the berries, there is only a tiny amount of maple syrup needed, which decreases the amount of added sugar in the tool significantly.

Bacon with eggs

• 1 banana

This recipe calls for 1 cup of coconut milk.

One teaspoon of vanilla extract

• 1/8 tsp. nutmeg powder

• 12 teaspoon ground cinnamon

One-and-a-half tablespoons of either plum powder or flour

• A dash of sea salt

Whole wheat bread, 8 pieces

RASPBERRY-SYRUPille

1 cup raspberries or other berries, fresh or frozen

2 tbsp. water or fruit juice

1 to 2 tbsp. maple syrup or sugar from coconut (optional)

France's bread-making industry

The oven should be preheated at 350 degrees Fahrenheit.

2 In a small dish, combine banana, coconut milk, vanilla, nutmeg, cinnamon, carrot, and salt. Stir until well combined.

3 The banana mixture is dipped into the bread pieces, which are then placed in a 13x9-inch baking mold. While they may overlap somewhat, they should not cover the whole disc bottom. Bake the bread with the last of the bananas. Work surface should have a light brown color after 30 minutes of cooking.

4 Top with raspberry syrup and eat it.

SWEET SYRUP TEE

In a small saucepan, combine the raspberries, water, and maple syrup (if using) and bring to a boil over medium heat.

2 Stirring and smashing the berries as needed, cook for 15 to 20 minutes over a low heat until the liquid has decreased by half.

Cinnamon and apple on a toasted bagel

Make two pieces of bread.

It takes 5 minutes to get everything ready, but it takes 10-20 minutes to cook.

QUICK PREPARATION FOR FREE KIDS 'FRIENDS

This is a simple, yet oh-so-delicious breakfast. In addition to regulating blood sugar and cholesterol levels, apples also aid to maintain gut flora balance and decrease fat and cholesterol. Anti-inflammatory and antihistamine characteristics of quercetin may be found in the skin of apples, which are significantly higher concentrations than in the flesh. Apples, especially the skin, offer a plethora of nutrients, making them a wise choice for your diet.

2 or 3 table spoons of coconut oil

• 12 teaspoon ground cinnamon

maple syrup or coconut sugar, about a table-spoon

A single, callous apple, finely diced

• Two pieces of whole wheat bread.

1 Mix the coconut oil, cinnamon, and maple syrup in a large bowl. Add apple pieces and cover with a hand mix.

2 Using a medium-sized pot, sauté the apple slices over medium heat for approximately 5 minutes until they are slightly softened, then move them to a serving dish. The same pan may be used to bake bread for 2-3 minutes on each side, if

desired. Apples should be strewn over the bread. Instead, you may raise a toast. Take a handful of the coconut oil mixture and rub it over both sides of each slice of bread with your hands. A 350-degree oven or toaster may be used to cook the oats until they're mushy and the apples are brown.

Blueberries and muesli in a bowl.

It's about equivalent to 5 mugs.

Time required for preparation: ten minutes

Preparation for youngsters may be done in a short time.

Because it has less fat and doesn't need cooking, muesli is a perfect substitute. Whole foods and p o r r o ISI s flakes may be found at health food shops. Add an extra two days to your sugar intake by finding the smallest m HCl r s components. It's a great workday morning alternative to oatmeal or drinks since it's both flavorful and filling. A variety of nuts, seeds, fruits, and spices may be found in these products.

Example

In addition to one cup of oats, you will also need:

1-cup dry grains like quinoa or oats, such as

Blown Cereal • 2 cups

- 14 cup of sunflower seeds

- 14 cup mantel

- 14 cup raisins

- 14 cup of dried cranberries

- 14 cup chopped dried figs

14 cup of unsweetened shredded coconut

- 14 cup of milk chocolate

• 1-3 tsp. cinnamon powder

CUENCOlle

• 12 cup of unsweetened milk or apple froth

Cups with a capacity of 3/4 cup

• 12 cup of berries

1 Shake the ingredients for the muesli in a dish or a bag.

2 Mix the muesli and the bowl ingredients together in a drawing pan or plate. 3

Breakfast with a movie and chocolate

Take two dosages at a time.

Cooking time: 30 minutes / 5 minutes preparation time.

Without the company of others, a gluten-free diet may be challenging.

Breakfast doesn't have to be unhealthy if you eat nutritious sweets. While quinoa is an excellent source of protein, you may use any cooked wheat, from oatmeal to brown rice, for your morning protein boost. Adding pudding to your diet is a terrific way to get your chocolate fix.

• 1 cup of quinoa

• 1 tsp. cinnamon powder

Milk without milk, 1 cup:

One cup of water

• 1 large banana

Boiling water with 2-3 tbsp bitter cocoa powder or locust beans

Almond butter, peanut butter, or seed butter, about 1-2 teaspoons

• 1 tbsp. linseed, hemp, or chia seed powder

- 2 tbsp of nuts

- 14 cup of red raspberries

1 In a medium saucepan, combine quinoa, cinnamon, milk, and water. Cook on high heat for 25-30 minutes, then reduce the heat to a simmer.

The quinoa should be mixed with the banana, almond butter, linseed, and cocoa powder in a medium bowl.

3 A serving of quinoa, pudding, and walnuts and raspberries should be served in a dish with a cup of boiling quinoa on top.

Soup with carrots and ginger

Prepare three to four large bowls

It takes 10 minutes to prepare and 20 minutes to cook.

Gluten-free and easy to make

Carrot and ginger soup is a simple, health-ful, and delicious weekday meal. Carrots' high beta-carotene concentration is still helpful for vi-sion, but antioxidants and other nutrients in car-rots have been demonstrated to protect against cardiovascular disease, cancer, and liver disor-ders.. Adding white beans, whether Cannellini or any other kind, gives the soup full of wit, robust, creamy, and rich in spirit white wit ego box wit to each of its individual components.

Extra virgin olive oil, about one-tenth cup

Onion: • 1 cup chopped

Ginger, freshly chopped, 1 tbsp

Peeled or rubbed and sliced, 4 big carrots are needed (about 2 cups)

• 1 cup cannellini beans cooked or canned and rinsed or other delicate white Papua

• Add salt to 12 cup of veggie broth or water

At least 2 liters of water

The following ingredients are in the following amounts:

1 In a large saucepan, heat the olive oil and cook the onion and ginger for 2 to 3 minutes until soft. Cook the carrots for approximately 3 minutes, until they are fork-tender.

2 Simmer for 20 minutes with the beans, vegetable broth, water, and salt.

3 Blend or mash the soup in a blender or with a dipping mixer until smooth. Serve at room temperature.

It takes 10 minutes to prepare and 20 minutes to cook.

Swiftly confirmation with little opposition to preparation so that you may drive fast without fear.

Soups like this let you use up a wide variety of veggies that would otherwise go unnoticed. No one ever complains about eating veggies because this soup is so good. The cream SC is so sweet and the coconut milk alcohol balances off the sharpness of the watercress. To make ® raw for this recipe, combine it with 2-3 normal meals, cook the onion just briefly before adding it to the soup, and let it cool completely before stirring it in.

- 1 tsp. of coconut oil

- 1 finely diced onion

- 2 cups of fresh or frozen peas

- 4 cups of water or vegetable broth

• 1 cup of chopped fresh cress

• 1 tablespoon of chopped fresh mint

• A dash of sea salt

• A sprinkle of freshly ground black pepper

• 34 cups of coconut milk. •

1 In a large saucepan, heat the coconut oil over medium heat. A few minutes after the onions are translucent, add the peas and water.

2 Then add the cress, mint, salt, and pepper after bringing to a boil. Simmer for 5 minutes with the lid on. 3 Add the coconut milk and stir until smooth in a blender or hand blender.

Beetroot and sweet potato soup

a total of six bowls

Cooking time: 30 minutes / 10 minutes of prep time.

Gluten-free food that's kid-friendly may be made in a matter of minutes. Enhancer of anti-inflammatory immunity

This potato and beetroot dish is simple to make and has a unique flavor. Sweet potatoes and beets make a flavorful and filling combo. To warm you on a chilly day, the soup has a pleasing beetroot hue.

• 5 cups of water or vegetable broth (if salted, leave sea salt underneath)

• 1-2 tablespoons of olive oil or vegetable broth

• 1 cup finely chopped onion

3 cloves of garlic, crushed

Thyme (fresh or dried): • 1 teaspoon

Pepper, 1 to 2 tsp.

Peel and chop two cups of beets.

4 oz. ground beef or ground turkey

• 2 cups peeled and sliced parsnips

A half-teaspoon of fine sea salt

Chopped fresh mint, 1 cup

• 12 avocado or 2 tablespoons of nut or seed butter (optional)

• 2 tbsp. balsamic vinegar (optional)

Two teaspoons of toasted pumpkin seeds

A big pot should be filled with water and brought to a boil.

2 In a large saucepan, heat the remaining olive oil and cook the onion and garlic for 5 minutes, or until soft.

3 Boiling water and salt are added to the thyme-infused peppers, beets, parsnips, and sweet potatoes. The veggies should be tender af-

ter approximately 30 minutes, so cover and cook for that amount of time.

4 Add the remaining avocado and garnish with a few leaves of mint (if used). Stir the ingredients together until they are well combined.

Using a blender or puree, mix in the balsamic vinegar (if using).

6 Place the pumpkin seeds and fresh mint on one side of the avocado slices and serve with the other.

Four bowls may be made with this recipe.

10 minutes of prep time / 15 minutes of cooking.

PREPARE FOR NEW INFLAMMATION WITHOUT GLUCOSIN

Miso soup is a classic Japanese dish made comprised of broth, miso, seaweed, tofu cubes, and onions, all served together in a bowl. Sardines and tuna are common ingredients in Japanese miso soups, yet they are regarded as herbs in our culture. We'll stay in touch, too. Soba noodles and azuki beans are purified and combined with the notion of chicken soup in a Japanese-inspired manner (Soba is usually in small packs and 7 ounces is about two packs in a typical package).

• 7 ounces of soba noodles (use 100 percent gluten-free buckwheat)

• 4 ounces of water

• 4 tbsp. miso

Drain and rinse 1 cup of azuki beans (cooked or canned), drained and rinsed

Some fresh coriander or chopped basil would be nice.

Two finely sliced shallots are required for this recipe.

Soba Stir Noodles may be cooked in a big saucepan of boiling water for around 5 minutes.

During this time, heat up the remaining water for the soup in a separate pot until it is just just boiling, and then remove it from the heat. Water should be added to dissolve the miso.

3 Rinse the pasta with hot water after cooking.

Serve the miso broth with the noodles, azuki beans, coriander, and chives.

big folded nuts into the pumpkin puree

Four bowls may be made with this recipe.

This recipe requires 15 minutes of prep time and 30 minutes of cooking time.

Quick confirmation without the need for veterinarian preparation and without the consumption of gluten

It is a comforting and pleasant soup that also aids in cleansing the body. It's delicious and filling, but it has the appearance of condensing books. For those of us who overindulged over the holidays and need a spiritual pick-me-up, this is the book for you.

• 1 small pumpkin pie, skinned, sown, and diced (about 6 cups)

Extra virgin olive oil, about one-tenth cup

• 1/4 teaspoon of sea salt

• 1 finely chopped onion

4-cup water or veggie broth

• 2 to 3 tablespoons of ground sage

• 2 to 3 teaspoons of yeast

Milk or 1 spoonful of peanut butter or seed spread and 1 cup of water or broth

• 14 cup of roasted nuts •

Peppercorns freshly ground

1) Heat the oil in a big skillet over medium heat and cook the pumpkin for approximately 10 minutes, sprinkling with salt for a light texture. Cook the onion in the pan for 5 minutes or until tender.

2 Cook the mixture after adding the water. As soon as you bite into a piece of pumpkin, it should be soft enough to scoop with a fork, so drop the heat to low and cover for 15-20 minutes.

sage, nutritional yeast, and non-milk non-dairy creamer Grate the soup in a dipping mixer or in a standard blender, and then serve it up..

4 Add roasted nuts and pepper to the top of the dish.

Pumpkin soup with grilled peppers

a total of six bowls

Cooking time: 40-50 minutes / Preparation time: 10 minutes.

Gluten-free food that's kid-friendly may be made in a matter of minutes. Enhancer of anti-inflammatory immunity

This soup's taste is enhanced by the sweetness of the grilled veggies. The art of vegetable cooking is in the time it takes to prepare the vegetables, whether it's in the kitchen or in the oven. Having a thick, creamy, and delicious non-dairy soup on hand is wonderful.

The following is the weight of one tiny pumpkin:

At least 1 tbsp. of olive oil

• 1 tsp. salt

As many as two red peppers.

In addition, there is a yellow onion.

• 1 clove of garlic

Water or veggie broth, 2 mugs

• 1 lime peel and 1 tablespoon of lime juice

Tbsp of Tahini per serving.

• A dash of cayenne pepper

• 12 teaspoon of coriander powder

• 12 tsp. cumin powder

• Roasted Pumpkin Seeds (Optional)

Set your oven to 350 °F.

2 Pumpkins may be prepared by frying them, cutting them in half, removing the seeds, then using a fork to puncture multiple holes in the flesh, if required. The flesh and skin should be rubbed with a tiny bit of oil, then sprinkled liberally with sea salt. Cook the remaining veggies in the oven.

3 If you don't want to chop your peppers, use the same procedure. Rub oil on the cut surfaces of the onion after halves it. Rub the naked flesh with the garlic tip and the oil.

4 Add the peppers, onions, and garlic after the pumpkin has been cooking for 20 minutes. Toasted pumpkin seeds on a separate baking sheet in the oven are also an option. Spread the veggies 10-15 minutes before cooking. Keep a close eye on them.

Take out the veggies and let them cool before using them. After piercing it with a fork, the pumpkin is very delicious.

If you have an immersion blender or a blender, remove the flesh from the pumpkin skin in a big pot. Add water, lemon zest, juice, and Tahini to a saucepan or blender, along with the chopped pepper, onion, and garlic cloves. Add the soup and adjust the liquid proportions to your liking.

7 Salt, pepper, cumin, coriander, and peppercorns are all good seasonings. Pumpkin seeds may be cooked and served with the meal (if used).

On weekdays, I eat tomato soup and chickpeas.

Take two dosages at the same time.

Cooking time: 20 minutes plus 10 minutes for prepping.

Warning: Wheat that is resistant to glutinitoniosis is readily available.

Cooking this soup is a breeze, and the result is a flavorful, rich, and satisfying dish. If you're looking for a fast weekday meal, this is ideal. Cooking this dish in a group of two or more can more than quadruple its yield.

- 1-2 tablespoons of olive oil or vegetable broth

2 cups of finely diced onions. •

3 cloves of garlic, crushed

- 1 cup of finely chopped mushrooms

- 1/8 - 1/4 teaspoons of sea salt split

Dried basil: • 1 tbs

- 12 tsp. dried oregano

- 1 or 2 tbsp. balsamic vinegar or red wine

• A can of sun-dried tomatoes

Cooked fat or a 14-ounce container of chickpeas (drained and washed)

• Two glasses of water

• 1 to 2 cups of finely chopped cabbage

1 The onion, garlic, and mushrooms should be fried in a big pot of olive oil for 7 to 8 minutes until they are tender.

2 Stir in the basil and oregano. Scrape the bottom of the pan with a wooden spoon after the vinegar has been added to melt it.

Tomatoes and chickpeas should be added now. Add water until the mixture is the right consistency for your needs, then stir until it is.

4 Pour in the cabbage and the rest of the salt and mix well. Cabbage should be cooked for 5 to 15 minutes, until it's mushy enough for your liking.

Plenty of chile.

Four bowls may be made with this recipe.

Time to prepare: 10 minutes; time to cook: 10 to 20 minutes.

In a hurry to make money

Soybeans have a wide range of nutrients that help decrease cholesterol and balance blood sugar levels without the need of saturated fat or ground beef. Coriander, which has a high concentration of iron, is also a good source of vitamin C. In order to get the intended iron, kt yellow, a distance of 14 of the necessary distance from the desired iron, kt yellow, is required.

• 1 finely chopped onion

garlic cloves, roughly crushed

• 1 or 2 tablespoons of olive oil, water, vegetable fat, or red wine

• 1 tomato tin (28 ounces)

A quarter of a cup of tomato paste or crushed tomato

1-quart dry beans washed and dried or 1-and-a-half cups for baking

• 2 to 3 tablespoons of chili powder

• 1/4 teaspoon of sea salt

• A quarter cup of fresh cilantro or parsley leaves.

1 In a large saucepan, heat the oil over medium-high heat and sauté the onion and garlic for approximately 5 minutes. Add the tomatoes, tomato paste, beans, and chili powder when the

vegetables have softened. Salt is a key ingredient in seasoning.

2 The more time you bake the better the results will be. As they continue to simmer at a low temperature, the tastes deepen and become even more delicious, much like the residue.

Serve with coriander as a garnish.

Lentil soup made with Indian red lentils

Four bowls may be made with this recipe.

It takes 5 minutes to get everything ready, but it takes 50 minutes to cook.

Preparation should not be a hindrance to your ability to drive quickly.

Spices such as coriander, cumin and turmeric are used to provide a robust and warming flavor to the soup. In order to prevent the spices and vihannesjuurina from grinding and making the s

m HCl's mind, add HCl to the sweet potatoes that

are already rich in vitamin A.

- 1 cup red lentils ä

- Two glasses of water

One tea spoon of curry powder and one tea spoon of divided or five coriander seeds (optional)

Coconut oil, water, or vegetable fat, 1 tsp.

- Cut 1 red onion into cubes

- 1 tbsp. freshly minced ginger

1 pound sweet potatoes, peeled and cubed

- 1 cup of zucchini slices

Peppercorns that have been freshly ground

- Sea salt

A vegetable or chicken broth or water, depending on taste.

Toasted sesame oil, about one or two table-spoons

• 1 bunch of chopped spinach

• Toasted Sesame Seeds

1 Cook the lentils in 2 cups of water with 1 tea-spoon of curry powder in a big pot. Simmer for ten minutes after bringing the lenses to a boil, or until they are soft to the touch.   2 Meanwhile, heat a large saucepan over medium heat, add the coconut oil and fry the onions and ginger until tender, about 5 minutes. Add the sweet potatoes and leave them on fire for about 10 minutes to soften slightly, then add the zucchini and cook until light, about 5 minutes. Add the remaining

spoonful of curry powder, pepper and salt and stir in the vegetables to cover.

3 Add the vegetable broth, bring to a boil, then simmer cook and cover. Cook the vegetables slowly for 20 to 30 minutes or until the sweet potatoes soften.

4 Add the cooked lentils to the soup. Add another pinch of salt, toasted sesame oil and spinach. Stir, allowing spinach to dry before removing pan from heat.

5 Serve with roasted sesame seeds.

This is a TCurry lentil patties.

Creates a dozen hamburgers.

Cooking time: 30-40 minutes. Preparation time: 40 minutes. Preparation time: 40 minutes.

Immune stimulant that is gluten-free and anti-inflammatory

A good texture that could be kept but was not too heavy was my goal when I first started making vegetarian hamburgers. I experimented with a variety of recipes before deciding to use carrots and a variety of spices to lighten the lentils. Thick and filling, these burgers are loaded with flavor and nutrients.

One cup of glasses with lenses

• 212 - 3 glasses of water a day

Three grated carrots.

• Cut 1 small onion into cubes

• 34 cup whole-grain flour (see gluten free options below)

• 1 12 or 2 tablespoons of curry powder

A half-teaspoon of fine sea salt

fresh black pepper ground to a fine powder •

Cook and simmer the lentils for about 30 minutes in a medium bowl of water.

Carrots and onions should be placed in a large bowl prior to cooking lentils. Add flour, curry powder, salt, and pepper to taste.

3 Drain the water from the lentils and then add the vegetables to the bowl after they've been cooked. Add more flour if you want the mixture to stick to the grater or large spoon. In order to get the right amount of flour, you need to know how much water is absorbed by the lenses and the consistency of the flour, so use it as a guide. Create 12 empanadas by removing a quarter of the ministry.

4Burgers can be baked or cooked. At the beginning of the sale, heat a large skillet over medium heat, add oil, and cook hamburgers for about 10 minutes per side. As long as you don't overcook it, you should be fine. At 350 degrees Fahrenheit, bake them for about 30 to 40 minutes.

Maple burger with a dill tang

Creates a dozen hamburgers.

Cooking time: 30 minutes plus 20 minutes for prepping.

Reflective amplifier for children

Vegetarian burger fun is what you decide to spend. You can mix and match the burger to the sauce to your liking. They go well with marinade, avocado, cherry tomatoes and lettuce.

• 1 red pepper

- 1 can of washed and dried chick peas or 2 cooked cups

- 1 cup chopped almonds

- 2 teaspoons Dijon mustard

- 2 teaspoons maple syrup

- 1 garlic clove, pressed

- ½ lemon juice

- 1 teaspoon dried oregano

- ½ teaspoon dried sage

- 1 cup spinach

- 1-1½ cups of oatmeal

Set your oven to 350 °F. Place a large baking sheet on parchment paper.

2. Cut the pepper in half, removing the seeds and stem and then place the pan with the cut side

of the furnace. Cook, preparing the rest of the ingredients.

3 Cook the chickpeas with almonds, mustard, maple syrup, garlic, lemon juice, oregano, sage and spinach. Press until everything is connected but clean. When the pepper softens slightly, about 10 minutes, add it to the oatmeal maker and press until sliced enough to create empanadas.

4 If you do not have a cooking appliance, mix the chickpeas with a meat grinder or fork and make sure everything else is chopped as finely as possible, and then mix.

5 Cut 1/4 cup portions and make 12 empanadas and place on a baking tray.

6 Place the burgers in the oven and cook until light brown for about 30 minutes.

Cajun Burger

Produces 5-6 hamburgers.

Preparation time: 25 minutes / Cooking time: 10-30 minutes.

ANTIPAL NUT GLUTE FREE

These burgers are made from grilled buckwheat (also known as porridge), which contains a routine flavonoid, contains plant lignans and is a good source of magnesium. All the heart-protecting nutrients in buckwheat can also help control your blood sugar. Combine this nutrition with incredible flavors. Turn them into a hamburger and get one of the best meals.

DRESS

• 1 tbsp Tahini

• 1 tablespoon apple wine vinegar

• 2 teaspoons Dijon mustard

- 1 or 2 tablespoons water

- 1 or 2 pressed garlic cloves

- 1 teaspoon dried basil

- 1 teaspoon dried thyme

- ½ teaspoon dried oregano

- ½ teaspoon dried sage

- ½ teaspoon smoked paprika

- ¼ teaspoon of cayenne pepper

- 1/4 teaspoon of sea salt

fresh black pepper ground to a fine powder •

- for Hamburg

- Two glasses of water

- 1 cup manna (roasted buckwheat) (roasted buckwheat)

- A pinch of sea salt

- 2 grated carrots

- A handful of chopped fresh parsley

- 1 teaspoon olive oil (optional) (optional)

MAKE A SECURITY

1 In a medium bowl, combine Tahini, vinegar and mustard until very thick. Add 1 or 2 tablespoons of dilution water and mix again until smooth.

2 Add the rest of the ingredients. Reserve the flavors to mix.

IN HAMBURG

1 Pour water, buckwheat and sea salt into a medium saucepan. Simmer for 2-3 minutes, then simmer, cover and simmer for 15 minutes. The buckwheat is fully cooked when it is soft and there is

no liquid in the bottom of the pan. Do not mix buckwheat during cooking.

2 When the buckwheat is cooked, transfer it to a large bowl. Combine grated carrots, fresh parsley and buckwheat sauce. Take a ¼ cup to serve and design hamburgers.

3 You can bake or cook burgers. Paistaksesi warm up a big pot over medium heat, add 1 teaspoon of olive oil and cook the burgers for about 5 minutes in the first days isell s page. C HCl nn s CAP s r and cook s still days 5 minutes. Keitt HCl skip to them, place them on a parchment lined baking-oven and bake at 350 ° F for about 30 minutes.

Grilled AHLT

He makes one sandwich

Preparation time: 5 minutes / Cooking time: 10 minutes.

Quick preparation without a child test

Give your BLT a healthy and delicious touch, replace bacon and avocado hummus. When grilling, the trade spinach was also a salad. If necessary, you can also use rubbed cabbage, rubbing it with your fingers until it dries and slightly moisten. It's the perfect place for a quick dinner with French.

- ¼ cup of traditional hummus

- 2 pieces of whole wheat bread

- 14 avocado cutlet

- 12 cup chopped salad

- 12 chopped tomato

To taste: • A sliver of rock salt

fresh black pepper crushed to a fine powder •

- 1 tbsp. olive oil, divided

The first step is to spread some humus on the bread. Place the avocado, salad, and tomato on one piece, season with salt and pepper, and then top with the second slice.

2 Add a spoonful of olive oil to a medium-hot frying pan before placing a cheeseburger in it. It takes about 3 to 5 minutes to boil the first half of a sandwich, and about 3 to 5 minutes to boil the second half, so keep an eye on it and keep an eye on it. Close the veggies with a spatula while using the spa.

3 To serve, take the pan from the oven and cut in two.

Pizza with a lot of black beans

assemble two 12-inch pizzas in the oven

Time to prepare: 10 minutes; time to cook: 10 to 20 minutes.

FAMILY STRENGTHENING QUICKLY The gluten-free resistance of family and friends

In addition to being very flavorful, this pizza is stuffed with a variety of fresh veggies. You may prepare it or experiment with summer-inspired items. Protein may be added to pizza sauce by using bean sauce. There are a variety of ways to bark in this situation. Simply buy two hazelnuts or a whole package, or make your own using Easy DIY Pizza Dough or Herbed Millet Pizza Dough and dividing it in half.

In addition, there are two ready-made pizza bases.

• 12 cup spicy black bean sauce

One medium-sized tomato, peeled and cut.

fresh black pepper crushed to a fine powder •

carrots, grated

To taste: • A sliver of rock salt

1 red onion, finely diced

• 1 avocado slice

Set your oven to 400°F.

Prepare a big baking sheet with two sheets of skins each. Each pizza crust should be topped with half of the spicy black bean sauce. Then, if required, add layers of tomato, pepper, and pepper.

3 Carefully sprinkle sea salt and sage over shredded carrots. On top of the tomato, layer the carrot and onion.

4 Bake the pizzas for 10-20 minutes, or until they are hot to the touch.

Slices of avocado and a third pepper should be placed on top of the baked pizza.

Pizza with hummus and other Mediterranean ingredients

assemble two 12-inch pizzas in the oven

Preparation time: 10 minutes / Cooking time: 20-30 minutes.

Gluten-free, kid-friendly, and a boost to the body's natural defenses.

This is one of his favorite meals of the week since it's simple to put together and can be served to a large group in a short period of time. Organize all of your previous vegetable-topped pizzas and then make anything you want. If you're not a fan of sun-dried and sun-dried tomato pizza, there are other options. Make it from scratch using Easy DIY Pizza or Herbed Millet Pizza Envelope and divide the dough into two equal-sized pizzas.

Zucchini should be coarsely sliced.

• 12 red onion, finely chopped

• 1 cup cherry tomatoes, split into two halves

• 2-4 teaspoons of chopped and chopped black olives

To taste: • A sliver of rock salt

Olive Oil Shower (Optional)

• 2 pre-made pizza crusts

• 12 cup of regular hummus or roasted pepper hummus

2-4 Tbsp of grated cheese per serving

The oven should be preheated at 400 degrees Fahrenheit.

2 In a large bowl, combine my cucumbers, onions, cherry tomatoes, and olives and season with sea salt. To keep taste and avoid drying in the oven, drizzle a little olive oil on top.

On a large baking sheet, place two skins. In order to cover each skin with herbs and cheese, apply half of the blemishes.

Bake for 20 to 30 minutes, or until the veggies are tender, depending on the thickness of your crust.

A mango and chickpea curry packet

There are three changes.

15 minutes of prep time

Preparation time is short since there is no kid test required.

The ideal combination of sweet mango and spicy curry, seasoned with calcium-rich tachyphyll. Make it for supper and pack the leftovers for lunch. You can also heat the veggies and chickpeas before packing them. Bring your own towels since the ones provided are a bit soiled.

In order to make this dish, you will need:

• 1 lime peel and 1 tablespoon of lime juice

curry powder, 1 tbsp.

• 1/4 teaspoon of sea salt

• 3-4 tbsp. of water

one 14-ounce container of washed and dried chickpeas, or one and a half cups for baking

Mango cubes, 1 cup

1. Inoculated and sliced red peppers

• 12 cup chopped fresh coriander

a total of 3 huge, complete tablets

One to two cups of green salad

Tahini, lime peel and lime juice, curry, and salt are combined in a medium bowl and whisked until creamy and thick. To make it a little more drinkable, mix with 3-4 teaspoons of water. You may also use a blender to get the job done. Salads should be seasoned to taste with plenty of salt and pepper.

add chickpeas and mango to tahini sauce along with pepper and coriander.

3 Place the salad in the centre of the packet, then top with chopped salad and wrap and season.

a box of falafels

Prepare six cakes and one bag

30 minutes for prep; 30-40 minutes for cooking.

This is NOT a toy for children's immune systems.

Combine the two of the world's most popular coffee specialties: falafel and hummus. Cook or fry the falafel instead of cooking veggies to give more nutrients to the falafel. Even though the recipe calls for six biscuits, making falafel takes a while, thus there are only enough biscuits in the recipe for six wraps. Alternatively, we can offer you some ideas on what to do with the falafel that is left over after everyone has eaten.

RATAKAT is a falafel

Cooked fat or a 14-ounce container of chickpeas (drained and washed)

• 1 grated courgette

2-chives, chopped

Chopped fresh parsley, about a fourth cup

Two teaspoons of black olives, smashed and chopped (optional)

• 1 tablespoon tahini, almond butter, cashews, or sunflower seeds

• 1 tablespoon of apple cider vinegar or lemon juice

• 12 tsp. cumin powder

1-fourth teaspoon of black pepper

• 1/4 teaspoon of sea salt

1-teaspoon oil of oregano (optional if fried)

package

• 1 pita or integrated package

• 14 cup of traditional hummus

• 14 cup of fresh veggies.

• 1 falafel cake cooked in the oven

• 14 cup halved cherry tomato

14 cups of cucumber cut up

• 14 cup guacamole or avocado, diced up.

2 tablespoons of cooked tabule or quinoa salad • (optional)

FILE A CREDIT CARD CLAIM.

Zucchini, shallots, parsley, and olives (if used) may all be processed in a food processor until finely diced. Don't remove anything; just push. Alternatively, grind the chickpeas in a large bowl with the grated and diced veggies before adding them.

2 Mix the batter with the lemon juice and cumin, pepper, and salt in a small bowl. Using a hand mixer or a pressure cooker, incorporate chickpeas into the mixture and thoroughly blend. Add extra salt if required. Form a six-span mixture using your hands.

3 You can make a cake, or you can bake it yourself. One tablespoon of olive oil and 10 minutes

of baking time on the first sheet are all that's required in a big skillet set to medium heat. Cook for another 5 to 7 minutes on the opposite side. At 350 degrees Fahrenheit, bake them for around 30 to 40 minutes.

package

Hummus should be spread out in the centre of the packet. Then spread the falafel cake out on the grass and smash it up. Toss in the quinoa, tomatoes, cucumbers, and avocados.2 Turn both ends and wrap as tightly as possible. If you have a sandwich press, you can press the pack for about 5 minutes. It is best to travel in reusable containers or reusable plastic containers.

1 Boil the medium saucepan with water and add the pasta. Keep the boiling point low, lower the heat and, if necessary, add cold water to continue cooking. Cooking takes 6-7 minutes, and occa-

sionally stirring to make sure they do not stick to the bottom of the pan. After cooking, use a strainer and rinse with hot or cold water, depending on whether you want a cold or cold bowl.

2 You can have raw vegetables so you can just cut them. To cook them, heat the frying pan over medium heat and fry the carrot with a little water, broth, olive oil or sesame oil. the carrot softens gently, add the pepper and toss the peas and shallots for a moment before turning off the heat.

3 Prepare the sauce by squeezing grated ginger to obtain juice, then mix or grate all ingredients in a small blender, adding 2-3 tablespoons of water if necessary to obtain a creamy consistency.

4 Arrange the bowl by starting with a layer of chopped cabbage or spinach (for spicy spaghetti)

or salad (for cold spaghetti), then sprinkle with other Tamar and then the vegetables.

5 Avocado chopped

CPSIA information can be obtained
at www.ICGtesting.com
Printed in the USA
BVHW091119270922
648083BV00013B/1351